The Complete Guide to 30 Sugar Free Days

Dr. Scott Olson ND
Wellbright LLC

CONTENTS

Welcome to the Guide

Welcome! You have quite the journey ahead of you!

The first thing you should know if you choose to go for thirty days without sugar or ***foods that act like sugar*** is that you are going to run smack into your sugar addiction and the (sometimes intense) cravings that come with addiction.

I will not lie to you; thirty days without sugar (or foods that act like sugar) can be hard.

The reason is simple. ***Sugar is an addiction***. And as addictions go, sugar is every bit as hard to break as addictions to alcohol, cigarettes, and drugs. Yes, breaking a sugar addiction is that difficult! Studies on sugar addiction show that it is very similar to other types of addiction and just as hard to break.

While all of this can sound bleak, it really isn't. Once you make the break from sugary foods, you will find you have much more energy, sleep better, feel better, and, yes, you will begin to lose weight (if that is your goal).

So while you are in for a bit of a hard time at first, the results are well worth it. By adopting a sugar-free diet, you are putting yourself on the path to much better health, as well as reducing the chances of heart disease, diabetes, Alzheimer's, and many other conditions that may shorten your life.

Eating foods I call "low and below" foods (I'll tell you about these later) is the best way for you to fuel your body for a lifetime.

And once you adjust to this way of eating, you will never go back.

Best of luck to you on your journey!

Dr. Scott Olson, ND

Foods that Act like Sugar

Keeping sugar out of your diet is easy enough to understand, but in case you haven't read my book, **Sugarettes**, let me explain what *foods that act like sugar* are.

Because I think the only way to be successful at keeping sugar out of your life is to stay away from sugar and the foods that act like sugar.

What are the foods that act like sugar?

There are many foods that act like sugar in the body. An understanding of these sugary foods came about because a scientist decided to test how individual foods change our blood sugar. The scientist would measure someone's blood sugar, feed them a specific amount of food, and then measure the change in blood sugar.

After studying thousands of individual foods and how they change blood sugar, scientists developed a measure of how these foods affect our blood sugar. They call that measurement **the glycemic index**.

They broke the glycemic index into three parts:

- **High-glycemic foods** are foods that can dramatically increase our blood sugar.

-

> **Medium-glycemic foods** are foods that have a moderate but still high impact on our blood sugar.

- **Low-glycemic foods** are foods that don't change our blood sugar much at all.

What the creators of the glycemic index are not telling you is that there are still other kinds of foods that don't show up on the glycemic index at all, and these are what I call "**Below the Glycemic Index Foods,**" and it is precisely these foods that you want to be putting in your mouth most of the time.

Actually, I will recommend that you choose foods that are either low on the glycemic index or below the glycemic index, or what I call "**Low and Below Foods.**"

All foods that are NOT low and below are high and medium glycemic index foods that act like sugar in your body.

On the list of foods that act like sugar are all sugars, all grains, starchy vegetables (potatoes, parsnips, and cooked carrots), and some fruit. I will have a complete list of both foods later in this program.

To summarize, the 30 Sugar Free Days Plan requires you to eat only low- and low-nutrient foods for 30 days.

Okay, that is the bare minimum. Let's get into a few more specifics.

What to Eat

The plan for the 30 Sugar Free Days is relatively simple: no sugar, no grains, and no starchy vegetables (potatoes, parsnips, etc.) or high glycemic index fruits (dates, watermelon, banana, etc.).

Put another way, you can eat most vegetables, a few select fruits, and almost any protein source you want, but nothing else. You also want to avoid any drink that has calories in it (that means no alcohol, no soda, and no fruit juice).

Important: At this point, I have to tell you that this is not necessarily a high-protein diet. Rather, I would like to see you replace all of your grains, sugars, and starchy vegetables with low-glycemic index vegetables or proteins.

One of the most common questions I get is: "How much can I eat?"

If you are typical, it is the sugar running around in your blood that has more to do with weight gain than the amount of calories you eat. I know this doesn't sound like what you are used to, but it is true. For most people, in most situations, calories are not worth counting.

The key to losing weight is to eat only low- and low-calorie foods. If you do that, then you can eat as much as you would like (within reason).

The Low and Below Foods

(Eat These Foods!)

The Low and Below Foods are what you want to eat during the program.

The "low" foods are those that have a glycemic index of under 55. Open your search engine and type "glycemic index for (your food)" to find the glycemic index for any food you are interested in.

The foods below are those that aren't even on the glycemic index because they don't change your blood sugar at all and are mostly meats.

You should have something fresh and crunchy at every meal if you can. Try low-glycemic vegetables, such as salad (any green), celery, broccoli, cauliflower, onions, garlic, cucumber, cabbage, peas, peppers, tomatoes, and others.

Most fruits are full of sugar and should be avoided. There are low-glycemic-index fruits you can focus on, such as berries, grapes, cantaloupe, and others (see below), but only use them in moderation. One of the most common reasons people don't lose weight during the program is because they are eating too many fruits. Fructose, the main sugar in fruit, is much easier to convert to fat in our bodies than any other sugar.

Meats, eggs, and dairy are fine to eat.

Some people who go on a high-protein diet will have that protein turned into sugar in their bodies, but this is rare. Dairy foods can also cause problems for some people. This makes sense if you think about it: dairy is a food designed to make small animals into bigger animals. If your goal is weight loss and you are eating a lot of protein or dairy foods, then you might want to consider cutting back on protein and focusing more on those low-glycemic vegetables.

The following list is not complete but will give you an idea of what you can eat.

FRUITS (RAW)

Apples, blackberries, blueberries, cherries, dried apricots, grapes, grapefruit, kiwi fruit, mango, orange, peach, pears, pineapple, plums, raspberries, and strawberries

VEGETABLES

Avocados, broccoli, Brussels sprouts, cabbage, raw carrots, cauliflower, celery, chard, cucumber, eggplant, green beans, green peas, garlic, kale, onions, jalapenos, peppers (green, red), radish, split peas, sprouts, tomatoes, lettuce of all kinds (green leaf, iceberg, red leaf, romaine), mixed greens, arugula, beet greens, collard greens, dandelion greens, endive, escarole, radicchio, red mustard, spinach.

BEANS

Baked beans, black-eyed beans, chickpeas (garbanzo beans), hummus (chickpea salad dip), lentils, pinto beans, red kidney beans, Romano beans, and soybeans

DAIRY

Remember: if you have problems losing weight on this plan, dairy is one of the first places you want to look. Full-fat cows' milk and most cheeses are on the allowed list.

Nuts and seeds

Almonds, cashews, macadamias, mixed nuts, peanut butter (no sugar), peanuts, pecans, pistachios, sunflower seeds, walnuts

PROTEIN

Beef, chicken, eggs, fish, pork, poultry, sausages, wild game

MUSHROOMS

All mushrooms, including Maitake, Reishi, Shitake,...

High and Medium Foods

(Avoid)

Stay away from all grains, including wheat, barley, corn, oats, rice, and rye. Try non-grains such as quinoa or amaranth if you need something grain-like.

Sugars of all kinds, including cookies, cakes, and candy, are hidden in salad dressings. Look for the hidden sugars in table sugar, brown sugar, powdered sugar, cane sugar, corn syrup, sorghum, honey, maple syrup, many juices, dextrose, turbinado sugar, amazake, sorbitol, and high fructose corn syrup.

Remember that you can avoid most of these if you are the one making and preparing your own food.

The following list is not complete, but it will give you an idea of what you should avoid.

GRAINS

All grains, including: barley, brown rice, corn, long grain rice, oats, rye, sweet corn, wheat, white rice, wild rice...

GRAIN PRODUCTS

All grain products, including: breads (all breads), bagel, baguette, blueberry muffin, bran muffin, corn tortilla, English muffin, Kaiser bread rolls, rice pasta, white bread, whole grain bread, Wonder bread, Remember, whole wheat doesn't make a difference; all breads act like sugar in your body.

BREAKFAST CEREALS

Cheerios, Coco Pops, Corn Chex, Corn Pops, Cornflakes, Crispix, Grapenuts Flakes, Grapenuts, Instant Cream of Wheat, Life, Quick Oatmeal, Raisin Bran, Rice Chex, and other cereals are all breakfast cereals.

Other Breakfast Foods

Croissants, cupcakes, donuts, muffins, pancakes, Pop Tarts, waffles...

Crackers and chips

all including: corn chips, popcorn, potato chips, pretzels, puffed rice cakes, rice crackers, soda crackers, and water crackers.

CAKES

All cakes, including: angel food cake

VEGETABLES

There are a few vegetables that you want to stay away from; these include boiled carrots, French fries, parsnips, and potatoes: baked, instant, mashed, pumpkin, sweet potato, and tapioca.

FRUITS

You want to limit the number of fruits you eat, but there are a few that you should avoid altogether: Banana, dates, tangerines, raisins, and watermelon

FRUIT PRODUCTS

When you process fruits, their glycemic index jumps up dramatically. Fruit Roll-Ups®, fruit juices, jams and jellies, fruit bars, fruit wraps...

Sugar and sugar snacks

All sugary snacks, including: candy bars, glucose, honey, jelly beans, sucrose, syrup, etc.

DRINKS:

Water should become your best friend on this program; avoid all fruit juices, all sodas, sports drinks, etc.

DAIRY

Diary is a food that I think you should be careful with (it is a food designed to make small cows into large cows; people who struggle with weight loss should avoid it), but dairy is low glycemic. Definitely avoid low-fat yogurt (the low-fat version has a higher glycemic index than full-fat yogurt) and ice cream.

BEANS

Most beans are safe, but you should avoid broad beans.

OTHER

If you have any questions about whether something is safe, just check the glycemic index (search for the glycemic index online). The foods you want to avoid are those that have a glycemic index over 55.

Here are a few foods that, contrary to popular belief, have a high glycemic index: Macaroni and cheese, pizza, popcorn, green pea soup, split pea soup

Meal Planning

The easiest way to stay on this diet is to go overboard with your meal planning. Yes, I said go overboard with planning.

Typically, if you are going to fall off of this diet, it will be some time when you didn't plan well and you are starving for something to eat.

Humans have moved from making their own meals to most of our meals coming from prepared food.

During this 30-day challenge, you are going to have to prepare a lot of your own food. While this can be daunting at first, it becomes easier the more that you do it. I suggest you make large batches of food when you cook so that something will always be within easy reach whenever you are pressed for time.

Remember that breakfast is your most important meal of the day, and especially so when you are on the 30-day challenge. Sugar acts like a magnet, and if you put something sweet in your mouth early in the day, then the rest of the day is going to be a struggle to keep from eating something else sweet.

The best foods to start off your day are fats and proteins, or something like beans, as they help you keep your blood sugar stable throughout the entire day.

Research has also shown that eating a low-glycemic breakfast actually helps keep blood sugar stable throughout the day.

If you are someone who is used to eating something sweet for breakfast, then allow your taste buds time to adjust to your new diet. You will be surprised at how sweet food such as avocados are when you keep the super-sweet stuff out of your diet.

Diet Tips

Here are a few tips to get you started on the program:

If you really want to make this a weight-loss program, you need to add exercise to your routine; it's as simple as that.

I'll say it again: You need to exercise in order to lose weight.

Fill your plate with either good proteins and healthy fats or a lot of low-sugar vegetables. Many vegetables are low-glycemic, and they contain plenty of fiber (which helps you feel full). Vegetables are also full of nutrients that your body needs (this also helps you feel full).

This is not a diet that limits calories. Generally, you can eat as much as you like. You will find that eating more often (every few hours) actually helps you with cravings and has also been shown to boost your metabolism.

I cannot stress how important moral support is for a weight loss program. If you haven't already, go find a friend (or enemy) to join you on this adventure. Create a support group or join one online. No one can help you more than someone else in the same situation.

The most important piece of advice I can give you is to not feel defeated if you make a mistake. Imagine that when you wanted to learn to ride a bicycle, the first time you fell, you stopped. I strongly believe that if you have learned anything in your life, you have failed your way to that success. Keep trying if you fall off the wagon. You will get to where you want to be. It just takes time.

Artificial Sweeteners

At first glance, artificial sweeteners look like the perfect solution to your sugar addiction: they contain no calories, and you can have your cake and eat it too.

The problem is those artificial sweeteners, while calorie-free, may cause you to consume more calories than you would if you hadn't eaten them, and they actually make your cravings worse.

The first thing to know about artificial sweeteners is that they do nothing to break your addiction to sweet-tasting foods. Sugar addicts are a unique group of addicts in that they want to stop their addiction, but only if they have a substitute. This is a little like recommending that an alcoholic drink non-alcoholic beer in order to break their habit. Most people see how silly that might be, but they still want a good sugar substitute.

What you need to know is this: continually eating sweet foods will keep the craving for sugary foods alive. This means that any tempting (real sugar) foods you run into (at the office, a birthday party, etc.) are all fair game—and out the window goes the reason you started using artificial sweeteners in the first place. My advice is to stay away from these fake chemicals.

It has also been shown that the use of artificial sweeteners can actually cause you to consume more calories than if you weren't eating them. The reason artificial sweeteners are causing you to overeat is not clear, but it may be enough to understand that your body does not like being tricked. Artificial sweeteners trick your body into believing that you are eating foods when you are not.

The most likely cause of overeating with artificial sweeteners is the body's insulin response. Your body's response to a sweet taste in your mouth is to release insulin. When insulin is released, it pushes blood sugar lower.

This lowered blood sugar may be the root of the reason you are more likely to eat more when you use artificial sweeteners: lower blood sugar means you feel hungry.

It is also good to know that almost every artificial sweetener has been a by-product of chemical experiments where the person doing the experiments accidentally tasted the chemical they were working with and noticed it was sweet. These sweeteners are the byproduct of chemical experiments and are not foods. These sweeteners are new chemicals, and our bodies don't know what to do with them.

We normally talk about the side effects of drugs, but artificial sweeteners also have side effects that range from headaches to diarrhea to neurological conditions (such as headaches) and a host of other symptoms. Aspartame alone was once the most complained-about food additive on the planet.

Worse than side effects is the possibility that many of these artificial sweeteners are linked to diseases. Saccharine may cause bladder cancer, aspartame breaks down in the body into methanol (a known toxin), and other artificial sweeteners are no better and are under investigation for a variety of disease connections.

Get rid of the artificial sweeteners in your life. They aren't doing much to assist you. Some people use artificial sweeteners as a smoker might use a nicotine patch. My experience is that this just doesn't work as well as you think it might. Everyone has their own path to a sugar-free life, and you might choose to try that for a while, but I think it is better to shun artificial sweeteners.

Coffee and Alcohol

CAN YOU HAVE COFFEE and alcohol? These are two of the most commonly asked questions when people start the 30-Day Challenge.

Let's take a look at each.

Coffee

Coffee is often a cause for concern for people who are looking to become healthier. In a strange twist of thinking, people think that something that makes them feel good should also not be good for them. While this is true sometimes, when it comes to coffee, there is good research showing that many of the phytochemicals in coffee are actually good for you.

The issue with coffee is one of degrees.

While one cup of coffee a day is probably okay, six cups of coffee is definitely not. Coffee is okay if it helps wake you up, improves your mood, or helps you finish that project. But it is not okay if it is the **only** way to make it through your day or if you are so hyped up that you are overstressed and not sleeping well.

What you are putting in your coffee also matters. Coffee itself is fine, but the cinnamon-mocha-caramel-sugar-ato is not (most drinks at Starbucks are 40 percent dairy, 40 percent sugar, and 20 percent coffee).

Coffee and caffeine can increase cravings, so watch out for that.

The take-home message is that coffee is fine in moderation without additives. I do prefer green tea over coffee, as it has a lower amount of caffeine and many more health benefits. I understand, though, that green tea may not be your...cup of tea.

Alcohol

You should avoid alcohol while on the 30-day challenge.

Alcohol is easily converted into fat in your liver.

Alcohol is a carbohydrate—and a simple carbohydrate at that. In many ways, it is just like the other simple carbohydrates you are avoiding on this challenge. But alcohol has another problem: it is easily converted into fat in your liver. This can lead to insulin insensitivity and a whole host of other problems.

During the 30 Sugar Free Days Challenge, you should avoid alcohol altogether and then test it and see how you feel when you start drinking again after the challenge.

Fats and Oils

Fatphobia is a very common part of our culture. Even with the popularity of diets such as Atkins, South Beach, Keto, and Paleo, people still shun fat.

The biggest problem we have is thinking that all fats are the same, which they are not. Fats come in all types and sizes. Some are healthy, and some are hurtful.

Most importantly, good fats are an essential part of our diet. We need fats just like we need proteins, vitamins, and minerals.

There is a lot of fat missing from most people's diets. Scientists call these fats "essential fatty acids," or EFAs. These fats are essential because your body cannot make them from other fats, so you have to get EFAs in your diet.

There are two types of EFAs that are most important for our health: omega-3 and omega-6 oils. While most people get enough of the omega-6 oils (found in vegetable and nut oils), they don't get enough of the omega-3 oils (found primarily in cold-water fish).

The problem with EFAs is that they are very sensitive to heat and exposure to air. This means that even though you are eating foods that contain EFAs, cooking destroys these sensitive fats. For most people, this means you need to supplement EFAs in order to get enough of these fats.

You can get your daily supply of EFAs by supplementing with fish or krill oil.

After supplementing with fish oil, you are probably wondering what other kinds of fats to use for cooking. First, you need to know that all the fats that you use for cooking are concentrated forms of food that are not found in nature (sound like some sweet substance you are trying to avoid for 30 days?).

Vegetable oils, in particular, would be very hard for you to obtain in large amounts if we didn't have our modern food processing machinery producing them for us. And vegetable oils are very harmful to your body—they increase inflammation and oxidative damage. Vegetable oils such as corn, soy, sunflower, or even canola oil all have a tendency to produce trans-fats and are usually produced at very high temperatures.

If you decide to use oils in your cooking, here are my suggestions:

- **Butter:** Yes, butter is a good and stable fat that works well for cooking.

- **Olive or avocado oil:** These oils are good and stable when heated and contain many benefits to our health.

- **Coconut Oil:** You can't use this for all your cooking because of the flavor, but it is a great stable fat that is solid at room temperature.

Menstrual Cycles

Many women have questions about what to do when their menstrual cycle approaches.

Women rightfully recognize that the premenstrual period is a very challenging time of the month. Cravings for all sorts of foods increase both before and during your period; this is when chocolate often looks like the only food worth eating.

While not certain, scientists suggest the cravings that come during the premenstrual period have to do with the loss of blood (and with the loss of blood, a loss of minerals and nutrients).

There are also extra demands placed on the body during menstruation, including changes in hormones that can increase cravings.

Many women report that being on a good diet (like a sugar-free diet) actually improves symptoms of PMS and cravings, but this sometimes takes a few cycles, so be patient.

As far as surviving "that time of the month," here is what I suggest:

- **Supplement**: A good multi-mineral can provide many of the missing nutrients.

-

Chocolate: If you simply cannot do without chocolate, try using carob or unsweetened cocoa sweetened with Stevia, or choose the highest cocoa content and lowest sugar version you can (above 80 percent).

- **Be prepared**: stock up on as many snacks that are on the "okay" list as possible.

With a little preparation, you can make it fairly easy; remember that this program is only for 30 days out of your life.

FREQUENTLY ASKED QUESTIONS

How HARD IS THE program?

Most people say that the program is both hard and not that hard. The first few days are the worst, and you might experience withdrawal symptoms, including intense cravings, but once you are through those first days, the program gets much easier.

As you start feeling better, you have more than enough motivation to continue the program. It helps if you have friends who are also doing the program at the same time.

Where do I find support?

The best support is the support you find in your local area. Find friends or family who would like to join you, or put up advertisements in community centers or churches asking people to join you.

What is the best way to prepare?

The first day of the program is called "Cleaning Day," where you go through your house and get rid of all of your temptations. It is also good to find someone else going through the program and meet with them daily or weekly to discuss your progress.

Do I have to eliminate all sugars?

There are different levels of commitment to the 30 Sugar-Free Days.

The first level is for the most committed, and it means no sugar or foods that act like sugar (all grains, starchy veggies, and some fruit). At the other extreme, people remove only *added* sugars. In between these two groups are people who eat whole grains boiled (like the way we eat rice) and foods such as sprouted bread or grains that are low on the glycemic index. People who continue to eat foods that act like sugar run the risk of feeding their sugar addiction (think how hard it is for a smoker to smoke only one cigarette a day), but it can be done.

The choice, of course, is up to you.

Any step you take to reduce the amount of sugar in your life is good.

The program is best if you can avoid all sugar and sugary foods.

Is this a low-carb diet?

Not specifically. When people first hear about a program to remove sugar from their diet, they think that they have to go to the other extreme: eating mostly protein and fat. That does work well, but people can also do the program by focusing on low-sugar vegetables and other proteins.

How much food can I eat?

You can eat as much as you want, as long as you stay within the guidelines of the program.

- No Sugar

- No grains (foods that act like sugar).

Don't worry about calories; read Sugarettes to find out why.

What is the best source for glycemic index information?

The best source of glycemic index information is this site: https://glycemicindex.com/

Click on the "Database" tab, and then simply enter foods you are wondering about.

Will I lose weight?

Most people who follow this diet lose weight. In fact, they lose a lot of weight. By aligning your body with what it really needs, you will automatically lose weight. If your focus is weight loss and you are having trouble losing weight, check the troubleshooting section below.

Breastfeeding Mother?

This is a healthy diet, and what is healthy for you is healthy for your child. Make sure to include plenty of fruits and vegetables, and make sure you are eating enough.

I'm a vegetarian; can I still do the diet?

Most vegetarians are actually "grain-arians" and addicted to sugar and foods that act like them and the rest of us. Vegetarians can do the diet; in fact, they may find it easier.

Protein in the diet is important not only for nutrition but also to keep blood sugar lower.

Specific Foods FAQ

Can I have Stevia?

The answer is yes (kind of). Stevia is an herb that helps with blood sugar control and appears to have no adverse side effects. A stevia extract was approved by the FDA for inclusion in food and appears to not have any adverse side effects.

Stevia has no sugar. It does, however, keep you addicted to having something sweet in your mouth (which can make you crave more sugar). I suggest using it in moderation.

Can I have honey, maple syrup, agave, or other natural sweeteners?

I get a lot of questions about sugars and which ones are safe to consume. Most of the questions have to do with finding a good substitute to take the place of white sugar. Sorry to say, but the short answer is that there are no suitable substitutes, either in natural sugars or artificial sweeteners.

Yes, sugars like honey, agave, and maple syrup have a small amount of nutritional value, but that nutritional value does not offset what these sweeteners do to your blood sugar levels. While people feel good about eating honey or other natural sugars, they are really no different from white sugar: honey, maple syrup, agave syrup, and so on, all of which act exactly like sugar in your body.

What about mayonnaise?

Yes, mayonnaise is allowed. You might want to check the label on the mayonnaise that you are using (it may contain sugar). You can find a pretty clean one at Whole Foods or other health food stores.

What about ketchup and mustard?

Popular ketchup brands almost all have a large amount of sugar (high fructose corn syrup), so they are not allowed on the diet. Mustard is a bit trickier, with some popular brands having sugar (either high fructose corn syrup, sugar, or honey) and others that don't. Check the labels.

What about peanut butter?

Peanut butter, along with almond, cashew, and other nut butters, is a great addition to the diet. These foods help us feel full when we are craving a sugary treat. The only problem is that most peanut butters have a lot of sugar in them.

It takes some getting used to, but natural peanut butter is easy to find at a health food store. You have to stir the peanut butter when you first bring it home and keep it in your refrigerator.

What about dairy?

Milk, cheese, yogurt, and other dairy products are allowed on the diet as they help to keep your blood sugar low, but there are two exceptions.

The first is if you are allergic to dairy. Dairy allergy is much more common than you might think, and I think everyone should spend two weeks without dairy and then reintroduce it to see if they are allergic.

The second is that you should avoid dairy products if you are trying to lose weight. Remember that dairy foods are intended to help small cows grow into larger cows, and they may do the same for you.

What about fruit or vegetable juices?

These foods that are stripped of their fiber act just like sugar in your body. Fiber is one of the great components of food that both slows down sugar absorption and makes us feel full. Avoid fruit and vegetable juices. Fruit and fruit juices contain fructose, which is much worse than glucose for your health and your waistline.

What about popcorn? Isn't it naturally low in sugar?

I wish I had a better answer for you than "that is just the way it is," but that is what the glycemic index shows us. We used to just guess what foods did to our blood sugar before we started using the glycemic index. We thought that brown rice would keep our blood sugar low and white rice would cause our blood sugar to rise. What we found out when we did the studies was that both brown and white rice caused our blood sugar to rise by about the same amount. It made little sense, but that's what the studies show.

Scientists suggest that there is something about popped corn that allows our bodies to digest it quickly, so it releases its sugar molecules quickly.

Special Diets FAQ

I'm an athlete. Can I really exercise without grains or sugars?

The best way to answer the question about whether you should eat grains is for you to test it yourself. I personally believe that grains and simple sugars cause a lot of the diseases we expect to get in our lifetimes: diabetes, heart disease, obesity, cancer, etc.

The 30-day sugar-free diet is not a no-carb diet; it includes fruits and vegetables.

I would say that you try the 30 days without grains or sugars, and when you finish, simply try eating wheat for a day, and you will know if that grain causes you problems or if it works for your exercise.

Having said that, people who are extreme athletes (those who exercise for over an hour at a time) have extra needs. While there is little research in this area, I suspect that eating a no-grain, no-sugar diet would actually benefit an athlete, but then you may need to make sure you are getting other forms of fuel during your long exercise bouts.

It is fairly easy to replenish the body's glycogen (quick energy) stores by eating a diet that has no grains or sugars. Many foods that contain natural sugars are on the diet, including fruits and vegetables. The issue arises when you are out for a long exercise bout and you run out of glycogen. Your body will then need to turn to your fat stores, or you will have to take in extra sugar when you are exercising in order to fuel your body. This is where you pay attention to your body and see if it is a problem for you and you lose energy (bonk) without taking additional sugar in while you are exercising. Most people can exercise for between 1 and 2 hours without needing to take on any extra fuel.

I'm a diabetic; can I do the program?

A diet that is free from sugar and foods that act like sugar can only benefit a diabetic and their blood sugar control.

Stopping all sugar, though, may lead to problems if you are on medication. I strongly suggest that you work with your medical provider to see if you can adjust your medication while you are going through the program. It is extremely dangerous to reduce the amount of sugar you normally consume in your body while continuing to take blood sugar-lowering medications. While the body is harmed by high blood sugar, this damage occurs slowly over time, but low blood sugar is a life-threatening condition, and you should monitor your blood sugar closely while going through this program.

Will this take care of my Candida?

This diet is a low-sugar and no-grain diet, and if you have Candida, you will certainly see your symptoms improve.

TROUBLE SHOOTING

WHAT IF I FALL off the wagon?

Understand that kicking sugar out of your life is a lifetime effort and that if you fall off the wagon, you can simply get back on the next day. It is good to know that many people have false starts until they get to the place where they are finally able to kick sugar altogether. Think of any other addiction and the struggles people have with it. It sometimes takes many attempts to have the tools necessary to stop for good.

What if I'm not losing weight?

Here are some places to look to see if you are having problems losing weight.

- **Are you eating fruit?** A lot of people turn to fruits when they start the program, but fruit sugar (fructose) is much easier to turn into fat than glucose.

- **Are you drinking alcohol?** Alcohol is even more easily turned into fat than fructose, especially beer.

- **Are you exercising?** There are guidelines for exercising throughout the program about exercising. Make sure you find some time in your day to get your heart rate up and get moving.

A small percentage of people convert high protein into sugar; if you think this might be you, consider adding in more low-sugar veggies (like salad greens) and less protein and see if that works for you.

BREAKFAST

RECIPES

BEANS

Breakfast, as they say, is the most important meal of the day, especially so for those of you going through the 30-day challenge.

Sugar acts like a magnet, and if you put something sweet in your mouth early in the day, then the rest of the day is going to be a struggle to keep from eating something else sweet. The best foods to start off your day are beans, as they help you keep your blood sugar stable throughout the entire day.

Research has also shown that eating a low-glycemic breakfast actually helps keep blood sugar stable throughout the day. The problem is that we are so used to eating something sweet for breakfast.

Here are a few suggestions and recipes that can help you get through the program:

- **Eat dinner for breakfast**: This is odd for many people, but it can work for you. It is surprising how quickly you can adapt to protein and vegetables in the morning.

-

Protein with vegetables: You can use a protein and add in any acceptable vegetables.

- **Smoothies**: Fruit smoothies, with or without protein, are a great way to start the day.

- **Eggs**: Eggs have gotten a bad rap. They are great for you. Try adding in some steamed vegetables, avocados, garlic, onions, or even mixed greens to make your eggs healthier and tastier.

- **Eggs and beans** are a traditional meal for much of the world. Beans have been shown to help normalize blood sugar throughout the day. Huevos Rancheros isa great way to combine beans and eggs.

When you let go of the notion that your breakfast must be something sweet, a whole new world of possibilities opens up at your breakfast table.

Breakfast Smoothie

Most smoothies are out of the program because they are just too sweet. Breaking up a food (as with a blender) almost always converts it from a low-glycemic index food to a high-glycemic index food. This smoothie, though, should be as low in sugar as possible because it is made with low-sugar berries and should fill the need for people to have something sweet in the morning. The fiber in the flax meal helps keep you feeling full throughout the day.

- 12-1 cup berries (blueberries, blackberries, etc.) in a blender

- 1-2 scoops of protein powder

- 12 to 1 cup water, almond, or coconut milk

- 1-2 Tablespoons flax or other oil

- 2 to 4 tbsp flax meal

Mix all ingredients in a blender and sweeten with Stevia (only if you have to).

Avocado Smoothie

Yes, you can make a smoothie out of avocados; just make sure that they are very ripe.

- 1 avocado

- 1/2 cup of raspberries or mixed berries

- 1 cup coconut milk

Blend all the ingredients together and serve.

If you really want to mix it up for an occasional treat, try using unsweetened cocoa (throw in a little Stevia if you have to).

Walnut Smoothie

You will need a strong blender to break up the apple and walnuts.

- 1 Apple

- 1/2 cup strawberries

- 1/8 cup flax meal

- Handful of walnuts

- 1 tablespoon flax oil

- 2 to 4 tbsp hemp protein

- Enough almond milk or coconut milk to blend

Place walnuts in a blender or smoothie maker and grind. Add the rest of the ingredients and blend until smooth.

Cranberry Smoothie

This is a simple, yet satisfying, smoothie recipe.

- 1 cup fresh or frozen cranberries

- 1 1/2 cups coconut or almond milk

- 1/4 cup raw cashews

- Stevia to sweeten (if needed)

If you are using fresh cranberries, toss in a few cubes of ice to make this smoothie cold.

Green Morning Drink

This is a refreshingly good morning drink.

- 1 large cucumber

- 4 kale leaves

- Half an avocado

- 1 tablespoon lemon juice

- 1 teaspoon powdered ginger

- 3 ice cubes

- As needed, use cold water.

Combine all ingredients in a blender or smoothie maker and blend until smooth.

Breakfast Chili

Chili for breakfast? You betcha!

- 1 can (30 oz.) tomato puree

- 1 (6-ounce) can of tomato paste

- 1 (4-ounce can) diced jalapeno peppers

- 1 (4-ounce can) of diced green chili peppers

- 2 (30-ounce cans) Pinto or Black Beans

- 1 (large) onion

- 2-3 potatoes, grated

- 3 stalks of celery, grated

- 2-3 cloves of garlic

- 2 teaspoons cumin

- 12 teaspoon coriander

- 12 teaspoon paprika

- 2 teaspoon parsley

Place all the ingredients in a slow cooker and cook on medium-high for 4 to 6 hours. Yes, this chili has potatoes in it, but the sugar in the potatoes is more than compensated for by the fiber in the beans. For the occasional treat, you can add an egg to this for your own Huevos Rancheros.

Apple and Kale Omelet

If you are going to eat eggs, make sure you surround them with plenty of fruits and vegetables.

- a few kale leaves (stems removed)

- 1 small apple or pear, finely diced

- 2 eggs

- Olive oil

- 1/4 teaspoon grated ginger

- Salt and pepper to taste

Heat the pan and add enough olive oil to keep it from sticking. In a bowl, beat eggs. Cook one side of the omelet, then add the kale and apple, then flip.

Chia Breakfast

- 1/4 cup chia seeds

- 1/2 cup almond or coconut milk

- 1 tablespoon almond meal (ground-up almonds)

- 2 tablespoons cocoa powder

- Sliced berries: strawberries, blueberries, etc.

Gently heat the coconut or almond milk, and then pour in the chia seeds. Allow to sit for 10-15 minutes, or until the liquid has been absorbed. Stir in the almond meal and cocoa powder. Add the berries and serve.

Mexican Breakfast

Serve this mixture in a bowl and avoid the foods that act like sugar altogether.

- 1 egg or a few cubes of tofu

- Refried beans or whole beans

- Sautéed onions

- Any other low-sugar vegetables that you enjoy

- Salsa to taste

Sauté the onions in a skillet, and then add in the vegetables. Add in eggs or tofu, and cook until done. Enjoy the contents in a bowl or on a tortilla.

Ful Medames

This is a traditional Egyptian breakfast; give it a try.

- 2 cups Egyptian fava beans, small

- 1/3 cup chopped flat-leaf parsley

- 4-6 cloves of garlic, minced

- 1 tablespoon of lemon juice

- 2 tablespoons cumin

- Chili-pepper flakes

- Olive oil

- Salt

Soak the fava beans overnight. Discard the water and wash. Bring the beans to a boil in enough water to cover, then reduce the heat and simmer for 2-2 12 hours (or until the beans are soft). Keep enough water in the pot to keep the beans covered. Stir in the herbs and oil. Remove two to three ladles of beans and mash them before returning them to the pot (to thicken the sauce).

Muffins

Muffins are definitely not on the diet. But these muffins, made with coconut flour, are lower on the glycemic scale.

- 1 egg

- ¼ cup coconut flour

- 2 tablespoons butter or coconut oil

- 2 tablespoons coconut milk

- ¼ teaspoon salt

- ¼ teaspoon vanilla

- (Optional) 14 teaspoon cinnamon

- 1/4 teaspoon baking powder

- 1-2 packages of Stevia

Mix the ingredients together and then pour into a lightly greased muffin tin. Bake at 350 degrees Fahrenheit for 15 to 20 minutes.

OTHER MEALS

RECIPES

OTHER MEALS INCLUDE SUGGESTIONS for lunch and dinner.

Here are some general suggestions:

Salad: Try mixed greens or straight lettuce salads. The benefits of these green foods are immense, but they also contain a large amount of fiber, which helps you feel full. Start every meal with a large helping of greens.

Grilled vegetables: fill your plate with vegetables and add a protein if you need it.

Stir-Fry Vegetables: Choose from your favorite vegetables, but you should also get a bit adventurous and try some that you are not used to.

Steamed greens: Chard, collards, kale, and other greens are powerfully good foods to add to your diet.

Soups, stews, and chili: Soups are another food that helps you feel full throughout the day. A study showed that having two bowls of soup a day helped people feel much more full and satisfied.

Chinese food: Most Chinese food fits the diet. Just avoid the rice and watch out for the sauces (many contain sugar).

Mexican food: Many Mexican food restaurants can keep carbohydrates (usually rice and tortillas) off your plate. Beans, meat, cheese, and vegetables make for a good low-glycemic lunch.

Here are some grab-and-go ideas when you are in a hurry.

- Fruit or celery with peanut butter

- Hummus and vegetables

- Fruit, dried or fresh

- Nuts and nut butters (almond butter, cashew butter, etc.)

- Plain yogurt (I prefer the non-milk yogurts like those made with coconut milk) with fruit

- Fruit-only frozen barsChoose the low-sugar version.

I'm not a big fan of protein bars, but so many people have asked me about them. I've relented and mentioned them here.

It is hard to find a bar that is sugar-free. There are low-glycemic versions of many popular bars that say "keto friendly" or something like that. Look at Larabars, Zone, or Powerbars, which don't quite fit the diet but are okay occasionally.

Avocado Salad

- Your favorite protein (chicken, beef, fish, etc.)

- Mixed greens or your favorite salad greens

- 2 medium avocados, sliced

- 2 medium papayas, sliced

- 1/4 cup toasted, chopped walnuts

- 1 cup of raspberries

Combine all ingredients and try covering with a dressing made of equal parts raspberry vinegar and olive oil.

Mango and Jicama Salad

- 3 to 4 medium mangoes, diced

- 1 small jicama, diced

- 1/4 cup chopped packed fresh mint leaves

- 2 tablespoons lime juice

- 1/2 teaspoon salt

- 1/4 teaspoon cayenne pepper

In a mixing bowl, combine all the ingredients and set aside for at least one and a half hours (or overnight). This salad can be eaten on its own or combined with greens and a protein.

Grilled Salad

Once again, choose any protein or vegetable you like. Here are some suggestions.

- Protein of your choice

- 1 small eggplant

- 1 zucchini

- 1 red bell pepper

- 1 small onion

- 2 tsp. red wine vinegar

- 14 tablespoon basil

- Olive oil

- Salt and pepper

Slice the eggplant into thick rounds and soak in a bowl of salt water for 20 minutes. Cut the rest of the vegetables into thick rounds. Drain the eggplant and mix it in a bowl with olive oil and pepper. Grill the protein and vegetables on a grill pan. Drizzle with vinegar and sprinkle basil over the top.

Bean Salad

This is a great summer salad. Choose fresh vegetables from your garden or local farmer's market.

- 1 small red onion

- 1/8 cup apple cider vinegar

- 1 15-ounce can of pinto or white beans

- 2 tablespoons fresh parsley

- 2 tablespoons fresh chives

- 1/4 cup olive oil

- Salt to taste

Dice the onions and drain the water off of the beans, then mix all the ingredients together. Add whatever is fresh to this basic mixture. Try green beans, broccoli, peas, or another garden vegetable. You can put the vegetables in the salad raw or lightly steam them before mixing.

Hummus and veggies

Hummus is one of the few mixed foods that have been tested and shown to be low on the glycemic index. You can now buy hummus at most grocery stores or make your own. You can also buy mixed-cut veggies at the store. Keep both hummus and veggies around for a quick snack or a good lunch.

- 16 oz can of chickpeas (also called garbanzo beans)

- 3-5 tablespoons of lemon juice (depending on taste)

- 2 tablespoons Tahini (sesame butter)

- 2 cloves of garlic, crushed

- 1/2 teaspoon salt

- 2 tablespoons of olive oil

Place all contents into a blender or food processor; use the juice from the garbanzo beans to make it smooth. Enjoy the hummus as a dip for any cooked meat and fresh vegetables (broccoli, carrots, cauliflower, and celery) you like.

Chicken of the Sea

This is a twist on an old chicken recipe.

- 1 can of canned or 1 cup chopped chicken

- 1/2 cup fresh dill

- 2 tablespoons lemon juice

- 1 tablespoon white miso paste

- 2 teaspoons of celery seeds

- 1/4 cup chopped celery

- Salt to taste

Combine all the ingredients. Serve in a lettuce wrap or on top of quinoa or another non-grain.

Roasted Protein with Asparagus and Green Beans

This is quick, easy to make, and delicious. My kids call the green beans cooked this way "green French fries."

- Protein of your choice

- 1 bunch chopped asparagus

- 1 lb. green beans, chopped

- 5 cloves garlic, minced

- Salt to taste

- Olive oil

In a mixing bowl, combine all the ingredients and spread them out on a cookie sheet or baking dish. Bake for 20-30 minutes at 350 degrees Fahrenheit. If you don't have fresh garlic, use garlic or onion powder.

Bok Choy and Shiitake Mushroom Stir-Fry

Bok choy is a wonderful green to add to your diet. It has a light taste and is packed full of nutrients.

- 1lb chicken

- 1/2 cup button mushrooms, sliced

- 1/2 cup shiitake mushrooms, sliced

- 3-4 cloves of garlic, minced

- 5-6 green onions, sliced

- 1 bok choy, chopped

- 1/4 cup vegetable broth

- 2 teaspoons fresh ginger, minced or grated

- 1 tablespoon soy sauce

- Olive oil

- 2 tablespoons sesame seeds (optional)

Grill the chicken with a little olive oil. Sauté the garlic, onions, and mushrooms in oil and soy sauce. Combine the bok choy and the rest of the ingredients and simmer or steam for 3–5 minutes.

No-Grain Noodles and Sauce

How do you make noodles without grains? Raw food enthusiasts are using carrots (see Ani Phyo's Ani's Raw Food Essentials) and jicama (see Lisa Mann's The World Goes Raw Cookbook), but I think the best is made from squash. Try any of the below combinations.

Noodles:

- Cut one medium- to large-sized spaghetti squash lengthwise and scoop out the seeds. Bake at 350 degrees Fahrenheit until soft (about 30 minutes). When you scoop out the meat of the squash, it looks like spaghetti.

- Zucchini: peel off the outer skin of the zucchini and then, using a vegetable peeler, cut wide ribbons of zucchini (to look like fettuccine). You may have to slice them lengthwise if you like a smaller noodle. Place your noodles in a colander and sprinkle with salt. Allow 30 minutes to drain.

Sauce:

- Choose any sauce you like, such as tomato sauce or pesto. We like garlic (lightly simmered in olive oil) and broccoli.

Serve with a protein you like. You can also add whatever you have around the house: nuts, tomatoes, avocado, asparagus...

Hoppin John

- 1 pound chicken, diced

- 1 medium onion, chopped

- 3 large tomatoes

- 2-4 cloves of garlic, minced

- 1 seven-ounce can of diced green chilies

- 1 can of chipotle chili

- 1 cup chicken broth

- 2 tablespoons cumin

- Salt to taste

This is a great "throw it all-in-the-crockpot and walk away" recipe. There is much more you can add to the mix, including carrots, peas, green beans, or whatever you like.

Cabbage Patch Stew

This recipe originally came from Lisa (a 30 Sugar Free Days partici-
pant), who added it to the Facebook page.

- 1 pound ground beef, chicken, or tempeh

- 1 chopped onion

- 2 Tablespoons olive oil

- 2 stalks of celery chopped

- 1 head of coarsely chopped cabbage

- 2 cups stewed tomatoes

- 1-15 ounce can of beans (any beans will work)

- 1 tin diced green chilies

- 1/2 teaspoon cayenne pepper

- 1 teaspoon of oregano

- Salt and pepper to taste

- Red pepper flakes to taste

Saute ground beef with onion and celery until lightly crispy (add a
little soy sauce for added flavor). Add the remaining ingredients to a
large pot and simmer for 1 hour, or place in a crock pot for 6-8 hours,
or until the cabbage is tender.

Cauliflower Soup

I like to make this a bit thick (just reduce the amount of broth) and puree only a bit of it, and then serve it over the top of quinoa.

- 1 large head of cauliflower, chopped

- 1 whole garlic bulb, roasted

- 2–3 leeks, chopped

- 1/4 cup raw cashews

- 8 cups of vegetable broth

- 4 tablespoons chives, chopped finely (to garnish)

Roast the garlic in the oven until soft. Sauté the leeks (use onions if you cannot find any leeks) and then combine all the ingredients in a soup pot and cook until the cauliflower is soft. Garnish with chives after pureeing all or part of the garlic.

Coconut Red Lentil Soup

- 3/4 pound of chicken

- 1 cup of yellow split peas

- 1 cup of red lentils

- 5-6 cups of water

- 2 medium carrots, diced

- 2 tablespoons fresh peeled and minced ginger

- 2 tablespoons curry powder

- 8 green onions (scallions), thinly sliced

- 1/3 cup tomato paste

- 1 14-ounce can of coconut milk

- Salt to taste

Wash the peas and lentils and place them in a soup pot with the water. Bring to a boil, then turn off the heat. Add in the chicken, carrots, ginger, onions, and curry powder; cover and let simmer for 20 to 30 minutes. Combine tomato paste, coconut milk, and salt. This recipe is best when you let it thicken up a bit, so allow it to simmer long enough to get thick.

Fajitas

While any vegetable will do for this recipe, I've included some that I think work best.

Grill 3/4 pound of steak or chicken in a pan with the marinade.

Marinade:

- 1/4 cup olive oil

- 1/4 cup red wine vinegar

- 1 teaspoon oregano

- 1 teaspoon chili powder

- 1-3 teaspoons of garlic powder

- Salt and pepper to taste

- Vegetables (choose any you like): Zucchini, yellow squash, onion, bell peppers (try red, green, and yellow), mushrooms (try portabella or shiitake), broccoli, cauliflower, and carrots.

Stuffed Peppers

Try using all different colored bell peppers (green, red, and yellow) to make this dish even more colorful.

- 1 pound of ground beef

- 4 bell peppers

- 1 yellow onion

- 1 red onion

- 2-4 cloves of garlic

- 2 stalks of celery

- 2 medium carrots

- 1/2 cup purple cabbage

- 2 cups of corn

- 1 large tomato

- 1 tablespoon lemon juice

- 1 tablespoon balsamic vinegar

- 1/4 teaspoon grated ginger

Chop and sauté ground beef, garlic, onions, and celery. Chop the carrots, cabbage, and tomato and mix them together with the lemon juice, balsamic vinegar, and ginger. Cut the pepper lengthwise and remove the seeds. Fill the peppers with the vegetable mixture and bake in the oven at 400 degrees for 25 minutes.

DESSERTS

WHAT ABOUT SWEETS?

One of the biggest questions I get is if chocolate is good for you and if you can have it on your diet.

Yes, chocolate is good for you, but it is actually cocoa that is good for you (most of the studies on the benefits of chocolate have been done on pure cocoa). When cocoa is manufactured into chocolate, many of the health benefits go away.

If you have a strong craving for chocolate, try taking a tablespoon of cocoa and adding it to your coffee. This experiment will let you know if it is the cocoa that you are craving or if it is the sugar in chocolate that you are craving. Cocoa plus coffee is very bitter, and most people won't like it, but try adding some milk substitute and a little Stevia and see if that helps.

These desserts push the envelope on sweetness, so be careful. I've included them for those times when you simply have to have something sweet but don't make them your daily fare.

Avocado and chocolate

As strange as this may sound, it is a traditional dish in areas of the world where avocados grow.

- 2 large, soft avocados

- 2 cups dark chocolate or carob chips

- 1/8 cup coconut milk, plus possibly more

- 1 teaspoon vanilla extract

- Stevia to taste

- Raspberries

- 1 tablespoon orange juice

Mix and mash this together and then eat right away.

Dark Chocolate

Here is another chocolate recipe for the diehard chocolate lover.

- 1 square of unsweetened chocolate

- 1 square of cocoa butter

- 1/8 teaspoon Stevia

- 1/8 teaspoon vanilla

- 1 teaspoon coconut milk

In a double boiler, combine the above ingredients and heat until melted. Pour into a mold or onto wax paper and cool.

Fruit Sorbet

The ripest fruits are the best. Pick two cups of each fruit you have available. Try these combinations:

- Strawberry and mango

- Cranberry and pear

- Berries and pineapple

Blend in a blender until smooth, and then freeze using an ice cream machine. Let it soften a bit before eating.

Banana Nice Cream

Remember that bananas are on the "avoid" list? So many people have asked to have bananas that I created this concoction. The coconut milk and almond butter slow down the absorption of the sugars, making this okay for the occasional treat.

- 2 frozen bananas

- 1 cup rice, coconut, or almond milk

- 2 tablespoons smooth almond butter

Blend in a blender or food processor until smooth. Serve right away.